I0423888

FREE BONUS!

5 MINUTES GUIDE TO LOSING 2 INCHES OF WAIST IN 2 WEEKS

THE 5-MINUTE FLAT-BELLY ROUTINE

SUPER FOODS & FOODS TO AVOID
FRUIT INFUSED WATER &
EFFECTIVE SHORT WORKOUTS

SUPERFOOD CORNER

APPLE CIDER VINEGAR

Action Plan : During your next visit to the Supermarket purchase Braggs Apple Cider Vinegar. Then Mix 1 tbsp (30mL) of ACV with approximately 8oz (150mL) of water and drink 3 times daily. Once on an empty stomach before breakfast, once before dinner and once 1 hour before bedtime.

There are many ACV brands around but it is important to take note that you should only purchase those with 'The Mother of Vinegar'. 2 This is cloudy appearance and is usually found at the bottom of the ACV bottle. 'The Mother of Vinegar' is a result of bacteria fermentation and is the most nutritious part according to most health advocates.

BENEFITS

-Helps with the digestion of protein and the breaking down of fat cells
-Reduces amount of time fat remains in the digestive tract
-Helps to regulate blood sugar (especially if you take it 1 hour before bedtime)
-Great source of potassium (80mg substituting with one ACV)

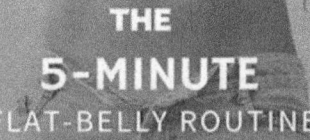

CHAPTER 2
FRUIT INFUSED WATER

3 Effective

Flat-Belly Short Workouts

CLICK TO DOWNLOAD NOW

https://weightlossprofessor.leadpages.co/5min/

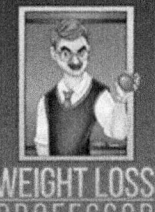

WEIGHT LOSS PROFESSOR

Copyright 2016 by Robin Houston - All rights reserved.

This document is geared towards providing exact and reliable information in regards to the topic and issue covered. The publication is sold with the idea that the publisher is not required to render accounting, officially permitted, or otherwise, qualified services. If advice is necessary, legal or professional, a practiced individual in the profession should be ordered.

- From a Declaration of Principles which was accepted and approved equally by a Committee of the American Bar Association and a Committee of Publishers and Associations.

In no way is it legal to reproduce, duplicate, or transmit any part of this document in either electronic means or in printed format. Recording of this publication is strictly prohibited and any storage of this document is not allowed unless with written permission from the publisher. All rights reserved.

The information provided herein is stated to be truthful and consistent, in that any liability, in terms of inattention or otherwise, by any usage or abuse of any policies, processes, or directions contained within is the solitary and utter responsibility of the recipient reader. Under no circumstances will any legal responsibility or blame be held against the publisher for any reparation, damages, or monetary loss due to the information herein, either directly or indirectly.

Respective authors own all copyrights not held by the publisher.

The information herein is offered for informational purposes solely, and is universal as so. The presentation of the information is without contract or any type of guarantee assurance.

The trademarks that are used are without any consent, and the publication of the trademark is without permission or backing by the trademark owner. All trademarks and brands within this book are for clarifying purposes only and are the owned by the owners themselves, not affiliated with this document.

Table of Contents

Introduction

I know that the title of this book is going to throw you off. I know a lot of people are going to be shocked by this book's title and they might think that it's wishful thinking. I'd like you to direct your attention to one central fact. The truth is losing weight is easy...on paper. In fact, it's actually quite simple: It's all about calories in, calories out.

To lose weight you have to do one of three things: eat less, move around more, or preferably both. If you do any of these, you will lose weight. How? It all boils down to achieving a net negative calorie state. When you eat less but maintain your normal activity levels, you have fewer calories coming into your system and your body will try to make up for those lost calories by burning up stored energy.

Animals, which include human beings, store energy in the form of fat and muscle. When you eat fewer calories, your body misses these calories. To be able to afford all its other energy expenditures it's going to compensate for these missing calories. It's going to start burning up fat and muscle.

Make no mistake about it, you're always burning calories. By simply reading this book, you're burning calories. When you walk around and breathe, you're burning calories. In fact, even if you're lying down on your bed, you're still burning calories because your body is pumping blood and breaking down the food that you ate earlier. Do you see how this all works out?

Consider your body as a factory. If you're going to do anything with this factory by making any of its machinery work, you need energy. Your body requires energy in the form of calories.

If you do any of the three things I mentioned above, you will achieve a net negative calorie state which would force your body to burn up calories. The more fat your body burns up, the lighter you weigh. Similarly, your body would also burn muscle for these calories. It has to get those calories.

The other approach, which is the more common way to lose weight is to simply move around more. You're eating the same amount of food but you're moving around more. Normally, people exercise to achieve this state. The same logic applies. When you move around more, your body's calorie requirements go up. It has to look for those calories somewhere.

Since you're not eating more to compensate for your increased activities, your body is going to have to burn fat and/or muscle to compensate for the calories you lost due to your increased activities.

This book teaches you a more passive way to lose weight. It teaches you how to eat less and lose weight. There is of course a trick to it. It's not a simple matter of just going on a diet. If that was the case, then you wouldn't be reading this book. All the existing diet books out there would work fabulously in a permanent way. Sadly, this is not the case.

It's all about passive weight loss

There is a way to eat less and lose weight. You have to go about passive weight loss the right way. This book spells out a winning strategy to go about doing that.

Chapter 1

You will fail if you don't have the right mindset

Did you know that the weight loss industry in the United States is a multi-billion- dollar industry? That's right, every single year, billions of dollars change hands in Americans' efforts to lose those pesky extra pounds. It never fails-each year, new diets appear along with new supplements and people go crazy over them. By the time the year is up, a new crop of products show up and people flock to those. This process goes on and on, and on.

In fact, the most recent sales figures in the global weight loss industry show that this worldwide market is in the billions of dollars. We're talking big money here. The reason why this is the case is because most people fail to lose weight. That's the bottom line.

They get on one diet or supplement; they achieve some results in the beginning then they get off the diet or the supplement and they repeat the process again with a new product or diet. If this sounds to you like people are on some sort of weight-loss treadmill that really has no point, then you would be absolutely correct.

The reason for this is actually quite simple. People fail in their weight- loss efforts because they don't have the right mindset. You have to wrap your mind around this central fact, otherwise, this book is not going to do you much good.

I decided to start this book out with this chapter on mindset because this is really the key to effective weight loss. Whether you are trying to start a new business, do well in school, achieve better relationships, or lose weight, whatever challenge you are faced with, you must have the right mindset for it. Otherwise you are only setting yourself up for failure.

I need you to keep in mind the following information, so you can have a game plan that you can fall back on to ensure success.

Starting is the hardest part

Sir Isaac Newton identified one of the most powerful laws of physics. When people take an action, they have to overcome a powerful force called inertia. Why do you think it takes a lot of effort to get a boulder rolling down a hill?

You have to overcome the initial resistance of that boulder. But once it reaches momentum, it rolls on its own. The same applies to your weight- loss efforts and pretty much everything else you wish to undertake in your life.

There will always be that stage of inertia. This should not come as a surprise because when we're trying something new, we're obviously doing something that we're not familiar with. It's new. It's something that we haven't experienced before. We may have existing habits we have to overcome. Not surprisingly, there would be all sorts of external and internal resistance.

Most people are afraid of change precisely due to the power of inertia. You don't know what's around the corner. You don't know how things will pan out. You have to overcome inertia by simply deciding to start.

A lot of people tend to give themselves excuses. What they would do is that they would gather information and think that they're actually acting on their plans. What they're really doing is they're kicking the can down the road. They're not achieving much of anything, but in their heads they feel that they are actually achieving something because they're gathering information, or in this case, reading a book.

I'm telling you right now, simply reading this book is not going to help you get rid of that extra weight. You have to start. You actually have to put this into practice. This is why it's really important to understand that starting is the hardest part. This is going to be your biggest challenge.

You have to decide to start on implementing the information outlined in this book. Simply whipping out your wallet and spending a few dollars on this book is not going to cut it. Everybody's doing that, but they're not getting any thinner.

You have to understand that it's one thing to think about losing weight and it's a completely different matter altogether to lose weight actually. Don't fall for the trap of thinking that by simply researching about weight loss you're doing something. You're just fooling yourself. You actually have to do it. You have to implement it.

The best way to get around inertia is to adopt the right mindset. If you're able to adopt the mindsets that I'm going to outline below, it would be much easier for you to start your weight- loss program. It would be easier for you to continue and finally scale up your efforts.

If you want to truly benefit from this book, you have to go through these different stages: Start, continue, scale.

Mindset #1: Assume that it is doable

You'd be surprised as to how many people buy diet and weight loss books thinking at the back of their heads that it's impossible to follow what's written in those books. They're always thinking at the back of their head that there's no way they will lose that weight permanently.

They know the drill. They know that when they try a new diet, initially they would lose some pounds, but as the days, weeks, months, or even years go by, they start piling all that weight back on. Worst of all, they even pile on more weight than they started with.

The reason for this is that they sabotage themselves mentally. You have to remember that if you, at some level or other, think that something is not doable, then it's not going to work out for you. The problem with weight loss is that people understand that it is possible in absolute terms.

They've seen the before and after pictures. They've seen celebrities dramatically lose weight. They know it's possible...for other people.

The problem is getting to the second stage which is to believe that it's possible for you. This is the big difference between theory and reality. In theory, a lot of things can work out but it only becomes real if we allow it to be real in our own personal reality.

You have to assume that this book is doable in your own personal reality. It can work not just for other people, but for you too.

Mindset #2: Starting low and slow is OK

A lot of people think that to lose weight you have to shed a dramatic amount of pounds, otherwise it's a bogus diet or the weight -loss program is not up to snuff. You have to get rid of that mindset. You don't have to start off your weight- loss efforts in a dramatic fashion. It doesn't work that way. Even small amounts are a step in the right direction.

You're only giving yourself an excuse to fail when you assume and expect dramatic weight loss. You don't have to do that. Don't sabotage yourself by thinking that way. Allow yourself to believe that starting low and slow is OK. Even a single pound lost is a step in the right direction.

Mindset #3: Enjoy the journey

Weight loss is a journey. It truly is, because you're learning how to tame your appetite. You're also learning about the level of self-control and self-discipline you have. It's not just a process of losing weight, but also a process of knowing yourself better. Look at it from this perspective. Relish the self-discovery.

If you go through the process and you focus on it, you increase the likelihood that you will get the results that you're looking for. On the other hand, if you start the process focused solely on a specific amount of weight that you will lose, you are setting yourself up for failure. You're so focused on a particular amount that you want to lose that you end up feeling that the weight - loss process is some sort of ordeal or punishment.

Mindset #4: Any victory is still a victory

Even if after several weeks, you lost only one pound, the reality is you still lost one pound. Do you see how this works? You're still ahead because you lost a pound that you had when you started. You have to define victory this way.

You should focus on sustainability. I know there are lots of diet books out there that make a big deal of the fact that people could lose 10% of their weight, even up to 50% of their weight. I mean, it's all exciting, but the problem is most of the people provided as test cases ended up getting all that weight back and more. In the end, focusing on dramatic weight loss only leads to defeat.

The key here is to declare victory once you have achieved sustainability. I'm telling you right now, almost all diet book in circulation out there do produce results, otherwise they won't get published. The problem is keeping the weight off.

One of the main reasons why they fail to produce sustainable results is because people who try those diets are always looking for dramatic weight loss. If they don't retain that drastic weight loss, they go back to their old habits.

You need to look at this situation from a different perspective. Focus instead on sustainability. A pound lost is still a pound lost. That is already a victory.

Mindset #5: Your weight is just one part of who you are

Truly sustainable weight loss systems are rooted in the right perspective. When people keep things in perspective, they don't beat themselves up too badly when they slip up with their diets. They understand that their weight is just one part of the many things that make up their identity. Always keep this in mind.

Don't feel that you have let yourself down because you did not lose easily the weight you wanted to lose. The problem here is when you get in an emotional downward spiral, you end up putting yourself in a position where you backslide to your old eating patterns. You put yourself in an emotional state where it's very, very tempting to engage in comfort eating. You start viewing food as a source of emotional assurance.

Don't engage in comfort eating. The best way to do that is not to judge yourself too harshly because of your weight.

Mindset #6: Hiccups and setbacks will happen

Let's get one thing out of the way right now. You will experience a day where you won't stay on this diet. That's perfectly OK. If you get knocked off the wagon, understand that this is to be expected. If you expect hiccups and setbacks down the road, then it would be much easier for you to stay on your diet. Compare this with how most people go about their weight -loss programs.

They think that their weight -loss program is such a slam dunk that they really get thrown off when they end up overeating for one day. It only takes a few more setbacks for them to get completely thrown off track and they abandon their diet altogether.

The better approach would be simply to expect that hiccups and setbacks will happen and it's perfectly natural. All it means is that you can go back on the wagon and try again. Since you allow yourself this flexibility, it's much easier for you to accept setbacks emotionally and you don't engage in comfort eating.

Adopt all the mindsets above so you can increase your likelihood of success. I can't repeat this enough: successful dieting is all about mindsets. While there are some mechanics involved, it really all boils down to what's happening between your ears. If you have certain beliefs, you increase your likelihood of success.

On the other hand, if you believe in the wrong things, and you have the wrong assumptions and expectations, chances are you will fail.

By adopting the mindsets I've outlined above, you pave the road for eventual weight- loss success. All this happens before you even start your diet. So be clear on the six mindsets that I have spelled out above.

Chapter 2

Losing weight without moving explained

I've already laid out the basic mechanics of weight loss in the introduction of this book. However, to make sure everybody's on the same page I'm going to go into further depth to make the case that people can lose weight without increasing their level of physical activity.

Focus on calorie suppression

As I've mentioned previously, there are only three ways to lose weight. This book focuses only on one method-calorie suppression. In fact, it's all you need. As long as you stick to calorie suppression, you will make progress. Ideally, you should increase your daily amount of exercise or physical exertion. However, even if you don't move around more often, you can lose weight. It's all about calorie suppression.

Passive calorie suppression

Passive calorie suppression is all about eating certain foods and adding them to your diet. I know this might sound crazy because a lot of people would think that a diet book is all about cutting away food or eating less. Well, this is how most diet books are presented. That's how they are positioned. That's also the reason why most diet books eventually fail the people who buy them.

You see, the human psyche is geared towards pleasure and runs away from pain. This is called the Pleasure-Pain Principle.

Human beings are animals and like any other animal, we're drawn to pleasure and we are repulsed by pain. When you add food to your diet, you are appealing to people's pleasure centers. This is pleasing to them. On the other hand, if you are taking food off the table or menu, you are creating a painful situation. People don't want to be deprived. This is why a lot of diets are often viewed by people as ordeals or punishments.

I'm telling you, it's no surprise that most of these books fail because people think that they are going through a hassle.

Passive calorie suppression is all about adding food to your diet while subtly cutting away portions. You still get to eat what you want to eat, but in slowly decreasing amounts. Best of all, you don't decrease the amount to such an extent that you end up feeling that you're punishing yourself.

This book is all about preventing people from feeling that they're depriving themselves. Effective calorie suppression mixes both passive and active calorie suppression.

End goal: What is your end goal?

The end goal of both passive and active approaches is the same. At the end of the process you are going to walk away with new eating habits. You're going to desire certain foods and they become part of your daily routine.

On the other hand, by adding certain classes of food to your diet, you end up displacing foods that normally pack more calories and make you gain weight.

This approach enables you to modify your lifestyle. If done right, it feels less like a diet and more like lifestyle change. Diets almost always fail. Lifestyle modifications, on the other hand, stand a higher chance of becoming permanent, which would you rather have? I thought so.

Chapter 3

Step 1: Slowly cut back on calories

The first step in the process of losing weight without exercise is to cut back on your calories. The great thing about this is that you can still eat what you want to eat. You can still stick to whatever food you currently enjoy. You just eat less of it. Also, you scale this step up over time.

This process happens gradually and it's very subtle. It is so subtle that it is not threatening. This is where many diets break down. They are so blatant, dramatic, and jarring to most people's systems that they end up upsetting people's normal eating patterns and lifestyles.

Now don't get me wrong, many of these diets do produce success. In fact, many diets out there produce really amazing overnight results. The problem is this weight loss is not sustainable. People can't keep the pounds off precisely because these diets are very threatening to the existing lifestyle of the people trying them.

As an initial step, you need to master the process of slowly cutting back the portions of the foods that you enjoy. The key here is subtlety.

By cutting back in little amounts, your body doesn't miss the food, and best of all, it gets used to the lower amount of calories, you then scale it down some more until you experience a net negative calorie state. As mentioned in the introduction, when you reach this state, you start losing weight.

Recommended program

You can pick and choose among the recommendations below. You don't have to adopt them all at once. You don't have to adopt them in sequence. Just pick the recommendation that is most comfortable and convenient for you at this time. What's important is you start with at least one of them and then follow the rest of the process so you can scale up. Feel free to experiment with variations of the suggestions listed below.

NOTE:

The 10% portion reduction mentioned below is just advisory. If 10% is too much for you, dial it back to 5%. Whatever the case may be, stick to an initial reduction that's comfortable for you.

Eat 10% less dessert

This is pretty straightforward, you just take whatever dessert you're eating now and just decide to eat 10% less of it. You can eyeball it. There's no need to do some serious calorie crunching or apply a calorie index. You can either look at the volume or the weight of the dessert. Whatever way you wish to do it, just start eating 10% less.

Eat 10% less snacks

Most people enjoy snacks. I'm not going to deny you your snacks. It's OK. You can continue to eat your snacks. However, do yourself a favor and resolve to eat 10% less snacks. Again, there's no need to do a formal calorie or weight count of the snack. As long as you can eyeball 10% less, you should be fine.

This doesn't have to happen all at once. You can start with 5% or even 3%. Whatever the case may be, just start dialing back on your snack consumption.

Eat 10% less of your main courses

For your main meals, start cutting back by removing 10%. Again, this doesn't have to be drastic. Maybe you can only handle 5% or even 3%. That's OK as long as you are cutting back some portion. What's important here is that you aim for sustainability. As long as you're consistent about the amount you're taking off, that's OK. The target of course is 10%.

Pay attention to your body

This is crucial. You need to pay attention to how your body is responding to your cutbacks. As I've mentioned above, you don't have to adopt all this cutting back all at once. You don't have to apply it across the board. You can start with one and then move on to the next item. What's important is that you have started cutting back.

Pick up on cues your body is sending you. Do you feel that your body is adapting quickly? Was it fairly easy for you to cut back?

On the other hand, is your body putting up a fight? Do you feel that 10% is too much? If that's the case, feel free to make some modifications.

If you're able to adapt to a 10% cutback pretty smoothly, then stick with 10% for now. Conversely, if you feel that you are depriving yourself or you feel hungrier because of the 10% cutback, you might want to scale down to 5% or even 3%. What's important here is that you achieve some sort of cutback while at the same time not inconveniencing yourself. You don't want to feel like you're depriving yourself or missing out on the food that you want to eat.

Get used to it

Now that you've determined the amount of food you've cutback, allow yourself to get used to this level. Whether you have cutback 10% or 3%, it doesn't really matter. What's important is you get used to that reduced amount of food.

Once you have gotten used to it, then try to slowly scale up. For example, if you're at 10% try to slowly scale up to 15%. Once you have reached this stage, scale up to 20%, then 25%.

The secret to this process is to do it gradually and comfortably. You don't want to shock your system by going from a 3% cutback to a 25% deduction. You can try, but I'm telling your right now you are probably going to fail. You would feel that you are on a diet or you're starving yourself, and guess what? You body's going to fight back. Worst of all, it's going to fight back by gorging on a ridiculous amount of calories. Don't put yourself in that situation.

Instead, find a very comfortable level and then scale it up slowly. The key here is to let your personal convenience and comfort guide you. You're still challenging yourself, but you're not pushing yourself to the breaking point. The way to do this of course is to simply listen to your body. Pay attention to your body.

Don't get all hung up on calorie count. Simple eyeballing or approximation is fine. Also, don't get caught up on pushing yourself rapidly. You're not in a race here. The only person you are competing with is yourself. What's the point of rapidly going from 3% all the way to 25% when you're just going to end up gaining all that weight back?

Focus more on enjoying the process and scaling up comfortably and conveniently while at the same time losing the desire to eat at your previous levels.

Chapter 4

Step #2: Slowly displace your food choices

As I've mentioned previously, there are two parts to this book's weight- loss program: active calorie suppression and passive calorie suppression.

Passive calorie suppression is all about displacing your food choices. Ideally speaking, it's all about replacing foods you normally eat that have high amounts of calories with foods that pack fewer calories. You still feel full, but your total daily calorie intake level goes down.

Why displacement?

Adding food to your diet produces better results compared to dieting because displacement is better than abstaining. With dieting, all you do is abstaining. Your system experiences shock when you abstain from certain foods or certain calorie level.

It's too much, too soon and it ends up with your body fighting back against you. You end up binge eating. Whatever progress you've achieved slowly gets reversed. Maybe you lost 25 pounds or maybe you even lost 50 pounds, but that will not matter because your body fights back so hard that you end up gaining all that weight back. Worst of all, you pack on more pounds. You don't want to put yourself in that situation.

This is where displacement comes in. Mentally speaking, you feel that you're still eating the same amount of food. But by making certain changes to your food choices and your eating schedule, you end up eating fewer calories daily.

Load up on water

Before you start actively displacing certain food choices, the first step is to load up on water. Water aids tremendously in dampening hunger. You see, your brain is always sending out satiety or hunger signals.

If your body is dehydrated, your brain is stressed and would send out more hunger signals. Technically speaking, you're not hungry but since your system is stressed due to dehydration, your brain is sending out the wrong chemical signals.

When you drink the right amount of water, this dampens hunger signals because it even flouts the satiety and hunger signals your brain is picking up on.

Water also helps because it distributes your nutrients better. When there's enough water in your system, the nutrients from the food you consumed circulate better. Your body, as a whole, feels less hungry and this reduces the hunger signals your brain sends out.

The net result is appetite suppression. You feel less of an impulse to eat. You can achieve this by simply loading up on water. What's important here is that you don't over drink water. Just get to the point where your urine is clear. That's a good test.

When you go to the bathroom and you notice that your urine is clear as water, then you are loading up on the right amount of water.

Load up on fiber

When you load up on high-fiber foods, your body feels fuller for a much longer period of time. The reason why this is the case is because fiber soaks up water. It also bulks up inside your system. It also soaks up nutrients and helps transport those nutrients in your bloodstream. When you put all these factors together, they lead to a longer and more pronounced feeling of satiety.

When increasing the amount of fiber in your diet, it's important to start slow. You don't have to get all dramatic about it. You can start by simply choosing whole grains for bread. Similarly with vegetables, you can select veggies with higher content of fiber.

If you eat a lot of potatoes, eat the potato skin as well to increase the amount of fiber in your diet. Again, it's OK to start slow. No dramatic and drastic change is needed.

Make it a point to eat high-fiber foods first

When you sit down for a meal, make it a habit to eat the high-fiber foods first. You're still going to eat your whole meal, but choose to eat the items on the menu that have high fiber first. By doing this, you increase the chance that you would feel full enough that you don't eat the low-fiber food items anymore.

High-fiber food items tend to be lower in calories and fat. This leads to a slow displacement right on your plate because high-fiber items make you feel satisfied enough that you cut back on fatty, greasy, or more calorie- dense items.

This plays out mostly on a mechanical basis. High-fiber foods are bulkier so they tend to take up more space in your stomach. This means you have less space for other types of food. As a result, your stomach sends out more satiety signals and you feel fuller longer.

Load up on low-calorie foods

I hate to be the bearer of bad news but the sad truth is there is no such thing as 'negative calorie food.' This is an urban legend. Foods that burn up more calories to consume simply don't exist. The good news is you don't have to shed tears over this revelation. Seriously, you don't. There are many low-calorie foods you can add to your diet to displace higher calorie items on the menu. As you get used to these foods, you overall calorie intake starts to decline until you can sustain a daily calorie intake level that is 30 to 80 percent lower than your normal intake.

I am going to list some foods you should consider. Pick and choose among them based on your taste and preference. There's no need to stress about packing as much of these foods into your meal plans. Add them based on your personal convenience. Don't stress!

NOTE: each item listed below has a calorie count per 100 gram serving. Please keep in mind that this 100 gram serving assumed no added sugar or oil or any other calorie-boosting ingredient.

Food item / Calorie count per 100 gram serving

Broccoli 34

Onions 40

Celery 16

Oranges 47

Watermelon 30

Kale 49

Brussels Sprouts 43

Beets 16

Tomatoes 17

Mushrooms 38

Carrots 41

Apples 52

Turnips 28

Cabbage 25

Zucchini 17

Asparagus 20

Grapefruit 42

Lemons 29

Cauliflower 25

When looking to spice up your food choices stick to the list below. These herbs/spices have a low calorie footprint.

Parsley

Mustard seeds

Watercress

Anise

Cayenne

Chili

Coriander/Cilantro

Cumin

Dill

Fennel seeds

Flax seeds

Garlic

Ginger

Peppers

Cinnamon

Cloves

Chapter 5

Step #3: Time to get mental

The way you select your food and the way you enjoy your food involves both physical and mental components. You see, certain foods give us a lot of pleasure because we attribute certain emotional values to them. There are certain foods that make us feel comfortable or assured during trying times.

A lot of people deal with depression by simply going to the fridge and whipping out a chocolate cake. Anything sweet reminds them, on a subconscious level, of assurance or of feeling comforted.

Food is not emotionally neutral. Be clear about this because the reason why you tend to gravitate towards certain unhealthy food items is because you associate them with certain emotional states.

When you were a kid, maybe your parents took you to get a slice of cake as some sort of reward. When you won an award at school or you got good grades, maybe your parents bought you certain foods that were loaded with sugar. This is as basic as parents rewarding their kids with lollipops.

You have to be aware of certain emotional associations you have with food and break those associations. If you want to modify your lifestyle and eat healthier foods while at the same time staying away from less than healthy foods, you need to be aware of these mental and emotional associations.

In this chapter, I'm going to step you through the process of consciously rewiring these associations.

What you're trying to accomplish

At the most basic, what you're trying to accomplish here is to associate the taste, look, smell, and texture of certain foods with negative mental states. I'm telling you right now, it's going to be quite difficult at first, but with enough practice you will get good at it.

You need to be able to get to the point where you can associate certain foods with fat. Basically, when you think of these foods, the next thing you will think about is the realization that, "If I eat too much of that item, I will get fat."

This may seem kind of basic at first but if you keep repeating this process, you end you retraining your mind so that you stop eating certain foods for certain emotional payoffs. You end up completely rewiring the emotional reward system that you have with certain food items.

What are the categories of food items that you should consider in linking with negative emotional states? You might want to consider the three food categories I will list below.

Salty foods

Salty foods can get quite addictive. Your body has been wired to crave certain salty foods for optimal water balance. This is hardwired into most human beings DNA. Unfortunately, salty foods also tend to be greasy and fatty. Fatty foods pack quite a bit of calories per gram compared to other foods.

By slowly associating salty foods with you gaining weight, you can go a long way in reducing your overall calorie intake. High amounts of salt in your diet also lead to water retention which also boosts your weight.

26

You don't have to dismiss all salty foods outright. You might want to start small. Just focus on the really salty items first and then scale up to less saltier items. Regardless of how you do it, get it in your head that salty foods lead to fat and weight gain.

Fatty foods

This should be quite self-explanatory. Foods that are fried or drenched in fat tend to pack a lot more calories. The good news is that not all fatty foods are bad for you. You can eat avocados, for example, which tend to be high in fat content and lose weight.

It's important to establish a negative emotional and mental association with fatty foods that are also loaded in salt and tend to be animal-based. I'm talking about fatty cuts of meat, chicken with the skin on, fried chicken, those kinds of foods. Also, greasy burgers and heavily processed meat-based foods fall in this category.

It's probably going to take a while to disassociate fatty foods from positive emotions, but it can be done. Just look at the end of the process. Just look at what eating fatty foods consistently and regularly would lead to.

I'm telling you right now, at first it's probably going to be quite challenging because fatty foods make you feel full and satisfied, but keep at it. Keep focusing on feeling guilty after you eat fatty foods.

Sugary foods

This is probably the toughest part of this process because most people have a very positive emotional association with sweet foods. However, there are two levels of sweet foods. There are artificially sweetened foods and there are naturally sweet foods.

Dried fruits are natural. Certain fruits have a high level of natural sugar and these are OK.

It's important to focus your firepower on artificially sweetened foods; constantly associate getting fat with donuts, cakes with a lot of whipped cream frosting. It takes some time, but it can be done.

The secret? Remember the guilt

If you've eaten a chocolate cake with thick frosting on it and it's loaded with sugar, it feels good at first. In fact, it tastes delicious. It's an awesome feeling. But once you realize that this meal would probably end up adding pounds to your weight, you start feeling lousy. You start feeling guilty. I need you to zero in on that feeling of guilt.

When you're trying to break positive associations of certain categories of foods with certain emotional states, zero in on guilt. Remember the tremendous amount of guilt that you felt. Remember how it felt when you were eating the wrong things and you were doing something wrong. Try to amplify that and link that to you feeling lousy about your weight.

Allow yourself to feel the high level of emotional intensity. Focus primarily on the guilt.

Tap into the power of visualization

Visualization is extremely powerful because it enables you to turn theoretical situations into something palpable and real in your mind. By simply closing your eyes and visualizing yourself at a certain place in a certain time experiencing a range of emotions, you can use visualization to break negative or unhealthy emotional associations with certain foods.

How does visualization work?

First, you need to budget at least 15 minutes of your daily time for your visualization mindfulness exercise. Take a break from your busy schedule and budget a 15-minute block of time. It's crucial that you exercise within the same hour or same block of time every day. This consistency increases the power of this form of mindfulness practice.

Pick a place where you can be by yourself or where you won't get disturbed. Close your eyes and imagine yourself in a different place. Zero in on the emotions that you are feeling. Paint a mental picture that triggers a certain range of emotions.

Visualization is a very powerful way to relax, and many people include it in their daily mindfulness practice. However, for our purposes, you're going to use visualization to help cement the negative associations you're trying to create between certain classes of food and a tremendous and overpowering sense of guilt.

I'm not going to tell you the exact way to do it because different people have different visualization settings that work best for them. However, whatever scenario you set up in your mind, you should focus on painting a scene where you are eating certain classes of food and this leads to you getting fatter and feeling lousy. Experience the tremendous amount of personal anguish and guilt you feel gorging on salty, fatty, and sugary foods.

How does it feel eating all those calories? How does it feel to eat food that you know will make you fat? You might also want to visualize yourself getting really visibly fat after eating these foods. Make sure that you experience a tremendous amount of emotional urgency.

Eventually, certain visuals would be closely linked and identified with a negative emotional state, like guilt, anxiety, and even fear.

The power of negative association

By constantly reprogramming your mind through your daily visualization practice, you would be less likely to eat foods that are loaded with calories. You would be less likely to have an unhealthy meal plan.

I'm telling you right now, this is not going to happen overnight. This will take quite a bit of time. However, you need to do this together with the other steps I've mentioned above. If you do them together, you end up losing weight sooner rather than later.

Chapter 6

Step #4: When you eat is as important as what and how much you eat

As I've mentioned in the introduction, your body is always burning calories. Your body needs energy. Even if you're just blinking or breathing, your body needs fuel for these activities. Any kind of physical activity, whether it's active or passive, requires energy.

The problem faced by people who have a tough time losing weight is that their metabolism works against them instead of for them. How? They often eat a lot of food at precisely the time of day where their metabolism starts to slow down. I hope you can see why this is a problem.

Since your body is burning less fuel at night, its ability to wipe out the calories that you have just ingested during night time meal decreases. Not surprisingly, some of these calories end up being stored as fat. Keep this up for a period of time and you're going to gain a lot of weight.

By simply choosing to time your meals a certain way, you position yourself to make your metabolism work for you instead of against you. There are two ways to do this. Feel free to modify these, but there are two basic ways.

Method #1: Eat most of your calories early in the day

During the typical day, your body's calorie-burning rate tends to be higher during the early part of the day than the latter part of the day. In fact, it drastically slows down come night time. It slows down even further past 7 PM.

If you change your daily eating schedule to load up on calories during breakfast or during lunch time, you end up matching your peak calorie intake with your body's peak calorie-burn rate. Accordingly, your body is in a position to burn more of the calories you ingest because of the timing of your meals.

If you follow the tips outlined in the other chapters of this book, you would have fewer calories to burn and you can achieve a net negative calorie state much faster and more frequently.

By simply loading up on a big breakfast or a big lunch and shifting your day's calorie intake to those meals, you end up burning more calories. With the right timing, fewer of the calories you eat make it to your waistline.

Method #2: Skip dinner

Now, this is more drastic. This method is really a form of fasting. When you fast, you simply stop eating. When you skip dinner, you end up increasing the block of time where you are not consuming any calories.

Most people already practice a form of fasting. This is called sleeping. When you skip dinner, you add a few hours to that block of time where you're not consuming calories. This can go a long way in decreasing your overall calorie intake and it can lead to sustainable weight loss.

The downside to simply skipping dinner is the tremendous amount of emotional blowbackmost people feel. I mean, let's face it, we're all creatures of habit and if you normally eat dinner, your body's going to put up quite a fight. However, if you're able to survive the first few weeks where your body is just simply trying to push you to go back to your previous eating schedule, this can pay off tremendously for you.

Experiment with both methods

I strongly suggest that you experiment with both methods and see which is more sustainable for you. Try to invest a few weeks to each method and figure out which is easier to adopt and leads to less resistance. What's important is that you pay attention to the signals your body is sending you.

Boost your body's metabolism passively

Another way to increase your passive calorie-burn rate without increasing physical activity is to just drink coffee. Coffee is a natural stimulant that speeds up the body's internal processes. Your body pumps blood harder. Your breathing pattern changes. This has a small but incremental impact on the overall rate your body burns calories.

By simply drinking a reasonable amount of coffee every day, you speed up your internal body processes which can lead to a net negative calorie intake. This of course will happen if you follow all the other tips outlined in this book.

Conclusion

Passive weight loss is not a theory. It is a reality for many people the world over who have kissed those pesky spare tire pounds good-bye... permanently.

By simply paying attention to the amount and types of food you eat, you can lose weight. Pair this with the right eating schedule and you can work with your metabolic system to boost your overall calorie-burning processes. Work with your body instead of against it and you'll achieve long-lasting or even permanent weight loss.

The great thing about the strategies I've outlined in this book is that you don't have to do them all at once. You can pick and choose. What's important is that you start to implement them and you're consistent with your efforts.

By simply sticking to whatever it is that you're doing, regardless of how low a level it is, you will get results. The best part is that these results would be sustainable.

Make no mistake about it, when it comes to losing weight, you're running a marathon. You are never running a sprint. Sustainability is the key. Even a permanent loss of one pound is a victory. Just allow yourself to scale up your results with time. I wish you nothing but success.

Thank you again for downloading this book!

If you enjoyed this book, then I'd like to ask you for a favor, would you be kind enough to leave a review for this book on Amazon? It'd be greatly appreciated!

Click here to leave a review for this book on Amazon!

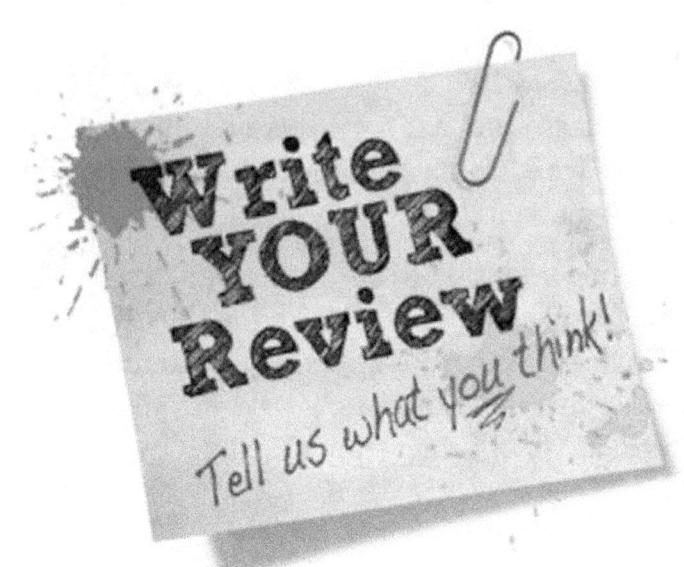

Preview Of 'Essential Oils Summer & Winter Recipes'

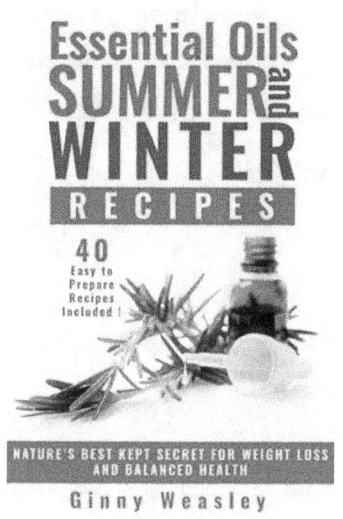

Introduction

Summer and winter can be harsh seasons depending on your lifestyle, at least for your skin. In winter, the weather is cold, dry, and unforgiving. In summer, it can be hot, humid, and very sunny. Most of us love to be out in the sun, sunbathing, and enjoying life. Yet, there are always the worries that our skin can be damaged by the sun. For those who gained the holiday weight and have not lost it during the spring, it is embarrassing to sit on a beach in a bathing suit. You no longer have to feel embarrassed or worry about the different seasons.

You have a guide at your fingertips that will teach you how to use essential oils, what not to do with essential oils, and their benefits as relating to your entire body's health, as well as weight loss benefits.

36

Do not worry anymore. Follow the recipes as outlined in the four recipes chapters, where you will discover 40 total recipes. There are ten specific recipes for winter, summer, weight loss, and overall health. You also have an extensive guide to learn how and why you should be using essential oils.

Click here to check out the rest of 'Essential Oils Summer & Winter Recipes' on Amazon.

Check Out My Other Books

Below you'll find some of my other popular books that are popular on Amazon and Kindle as well. Simply click on the links below to check them out. Alternatively, you can visit my author page on Amazon to see other works published by me.

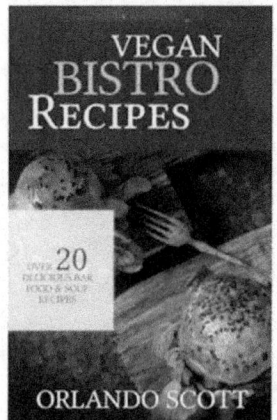 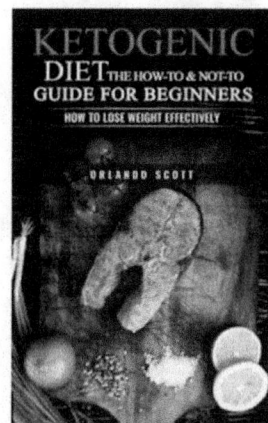 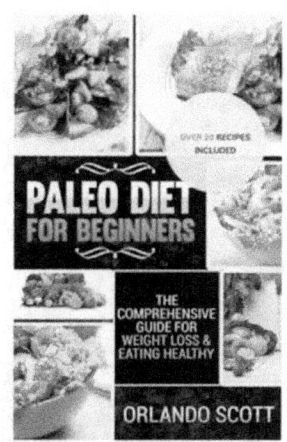

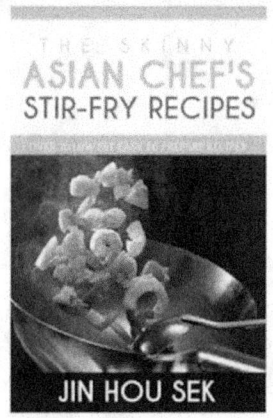 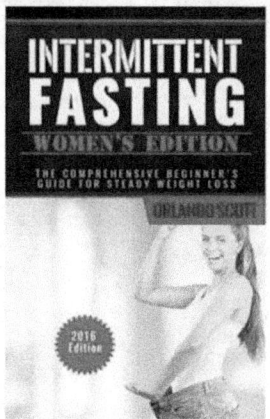

Vegan Bistro Recipes Link

Ketogenic Diet Link

Paleo Diet For Beginners Link

<u>The Skinny Asian Chef's Stir-Fry Recipes Link</u>

<u>Intermittent Fasting Women's Edition Link</u>

If the links do not work, for whatever reason, you can simply search for these titles on the Amazon website to find them.

www.ingramcontent.com/pod-product-compliance
Lightning Source LLC
Chambersburg PA
CBHW061801280526
45787CB00003BA/1434